Lavender

Uncover The Incredible Health And Beauty Uses You Are Missing From This Easy To Grow Relaxing Flower

Written By
Ashley Stone

Ashley Stone

© **Copyright 2020 by Ashley Stone - All rights reserved.**

This document is geared towards providing exact and reliable information in regards to the topic and issue covered. The publication is sold with the idea that the publisher is not required to render accounting, officially permitted, or otherwise, qualified services. If advice is necessary, legal or professional, a practiced individual in the profession should be ordered.

- From a Declaration of Principles which was accepted and approved equally by a Committee of the American Bar Association and a Committee of Publishers and Associations.

In no way is it legal to reproduce, duplicate, or transmit any part of this document in either electronic means or in printed format. Recording of this publication is strictly prohibited and any storage of this document is not allowed unless with written permission from the publisher. All rights reserved.

The information provided herein is stated to be truthful and consistent, in that any liability, in terms of inattention or otherwise, by any usage or abuse of any policies, processes, or directions contained within is the solitary and utter responsibility of the recipient reader. Under no circumstances will any legal responsibility or blame be held against the publisher for any reparation, damages, or monetary loss due to the information herein, either directly or indirectly.

Respective authors own all copyrights not held by the publisher.

The information herein is offered for informational purposes solely, and is universal as so. The presentation of the information is without contract or any type of guarantee assurance.

The trademarks that are used are without any consent, and the publication of the trademark is without permission or backing by the trademark owner. All trademarks and brands within this book are for clarifying purposes only and are the owned by the owners themselves, not affiliated with this document.

Table of Contents

Introduction 7

Chapter 1 8

Lavender, the "Forgotten" Herb 8

    The Ultimate Healing Herb? 9

    Cooking with Lavender? 10

Chapter 2 12

Growing Lavender 12

    Growing Instructions in Soil 12

    Growing in Pots and Planters 13

    Harvesting Lavender 15

Chapter 3 17

Lavender for Healing 17

    Muscle Strain Relief 20

    Coughs, Colds and Chest Problems 20

    Skin Conditions and Acne 21

    Sprains and Strains 21

    Stings and Scratches 21

    Burns and Sunburn 22

    Alopecia Areata 22

    Dried Lavender Uses 22

    Lavender Salve 23

    Safety Notes 24

    Interactions with antidepressants 24

    Allergic Reactions 25

    Pregnant and Breastfeeding Women 25

    Children and Lavender 25

Chapter 4 26

Preserving Lavender 26

    Drying Lavender 26

    Distilling Lavender Essential Oil 28

    Infused Lavender Oil 30

Chapter 5 32

Cooking with Lavender 32

    Simple Lavender Cookery Tricks 33

    Smoked Salmon with Lavender and Dill 34

Pork or Lamb with Lavender..34

Wine and Lavender Sauce 34

Tuna Steaks with Lavender and Herb Crust 35

Lavender Stews 35

Creme Brulee with Lavender 36

Lavender Shortbread 37

Conclusion 39

Introduction

I want to thank you and congratulate you for buying the book, "Lavender, Beyond the Garden".

This book contains proven steps and strategies on how to make the most of this much over-looked plant. With information on how to use Lavender for cookery and for its medicinal qualities, this book contains a wealth of information on a herb that has a long history and a surprising variety of uses!

Thanks again for buying this book, I hope you enjoy it!

Chapter 1

Lavender, the "Forgotten" Herb

Herbs have been used for several thousand years in both food and medicinal settings. Of all herbs, one in particular stands out; Lavender. A member of the mint family, this highly scented flowering plant is perhaps the most beautiful and most versatile of "herbs". In many gardens today it is simply grown for its rich purple coloring and its heavy, distinctive scent. However, the plant has some very special qualities which make it a valuable commodity and vast fields of lavender are commercially farmed for use in the scent and cosmetic industries.

Lavender and humans go back a long way; the ancient Greek name is "Nardus" - the name stemming from the Syrian city of Naarda. In ancient times it was a key ingredient in incense and the plant was considered sacred in many cultures. It was widely used to create scented oils used in ritual and is even mentioned in the Bible in the Song of Solomon.

By Roman times the name we all recognize today was established and, tellingly, the word Lavender is linked to the word 'lavare' – the Latin for "to wash". The plant is widespread in the wild across the Mediterranean and has been cultivated in that region for at least two thousand years. Hardy, resistant to drought and easy to care for the popularity of Lavender as both a garden plant and a commercially farmed herb has seen it spread across the world to many different countries.

Most large-scale commercial producers of Lavender farm the plant to extract essential oils which are then used in soaps, scents and other cosmetics. The flowers from the plant can also be used and these are often found in pillows or sachets and, of course, Lavender is an essential ingredient in potpourri. Lavender has been widely used in medical settings in the past – and is a particularly popular ingredient in Chinese medicine. In the West a move away from traditional methods of healing has seen Lavender's popularity as a medicinal herb decline to some extent. In recent years, however, this trend has reversed as an interest has developed in forgotten, traditional remedies using the natural healing qualities of plants and herbs.

The Ultimate Healing Herb?

Most herbs have a range of beneficial medicinal qualities that have been recognized within traditional medicine for thousands of years, and lavender is no exception. Unlike modern pills and potions, many herbal remedies contain natural, organic produce and for this reason alone a widespread interest in their use has developed in the last forty or so years. Lavender, in particular, is known for its antiseptic, anti-inflammatory and disinfectant qualities. Used topically on the skin it has been shown to ease small burns, bites, cuts and grazes and is also believed to be useful as an acne treatment. Lavender oil can also be used to treat indigestion and heartburn, while both the oil and flowers can help to reduce nausea and headaches. Lavender also has been regarded for many years as a relaxing herb which aids healthy sleep. In recent years some small academic studies have been undertaken which appear to support this fact. Both anxiety and insomnia seem to be positively affected by the use of Lavender and using a Lavender pillow (or scent) seems to reduce insomnia and promote deeper, healthier sleep. Studies have also been conducted on the effects of Lavender on eczema and alopecia (hair loss caused by an autoimmune disease) and both have shown positive results – although the test groups have been small and further studies may be needed to confirm the results.

Cooking with Lavender?

Unlike many other herbs Lavender has somewhat fallen out of favor in terms of culinary use; it has however a long history of use as a flavoring and seasoning for both sweet and savory dishes. It's the latter that has particularly fallen out of favor, perhaps, but many traditional culinary uses for lavender deserve a closer look!

Creating a floral, slightly sweet flavor, lavender can be used in soups, stews, salads, seafood dishes, cakes, pastries and confectionery. The flowers of the plant contain the essential oils, and therefore the strongest flavor, but the leaves or stalk can also provide flavor in a dish and may be most suitable in savory dishes – giving a more subtle hint of the flavor.

This book explores the main medicinal uses of Lavender and introduces you to some of the more unusual uses Lavender can be put to in the home as well as in the kitchen! Dried Lavender and essential oil can be purchased but Lavender is an easy plant to cultivate in your own garden (or in pots) and before we look more fully at the uses of Lavender, we'll take a look in the next chapter at the essentials of growing Lavender.

Chapter 2

Growing Lavender

Lavender is a Mediterranean plant but that doesn't mean you have to live in a Mediterranean climate to grow it! The plant is, in fact, hardy and adaptable. The arid conditions of the Mediterranean, with low rainfall, mean that the plant is also one that thrives in poor soil conditions and is not a high maintenance plant – making it ideal for those who are less than green-fingered! The plant will survive well in a sunny spot in most gardens and can be grown in a border or in planters or pots.

Growing Instructions in Soil

Lavender is usually planted between April and May – normally outside of these times it will not establish well. A slow growing plant, it prefers chalk or alkaline soils and will cope well in relatively poor soil in which other plants may struggle. Drainage is important – remember lavender in the wild thrives on well drained rocky hillsides – and waterlogged ground will, at best, see poor growth and, more likely, no growth. In thick, clay based soils Lavender will do less well. In these conditions it's best to add gravel and some organic matter – creating a mound of organic compost and gravel, if possible, will create the best conditions for Lavender in clay soils. Again, ensure that water can flow away from the roots for best results.

Lavender loves sun! Full sun positions are the best for the plant, if possible, although partial sun conditions should be enough to establish a healthy shrub. Shaded or low sun areas should be avoided as this will not provide the amount of light that lavender needs to thrive. Tolerant to drought, Lavender will do well in sea-side locations and is a perfect (low maintenance) plant for gravel gardens (also low maintenance!). Plants should be spaced around 45-90cm (18-36in) apart, if you're planting amongst other types of plan. In this case plant 3-4 lavender plants together to create a good group. If you're planting Lavender on its own, spacing should be reduced to about 40-50cms (1ft-16in). For a Lavender hedge (an attractive and highly scented border) use the same spacing.

Growing in Pots and Planters

Lavender is a shrub-like plant and requires reasonably large pots and planters. The structure of the plant, the color and scent all make it an attractive addition to any garden, porch or yard. Lavender likes relatively constricted conditions for its roots – so pots should be chosen that allow the root-ball to fill much of the space. For full sized shrubs pots should be 30-40 cm (1ft – 16inches) in diameter. A multipurpose compost is best and add gravel and grit to a ratio of about 30% for best results. Slow release fertilizer should be added to the mixture to provide adequate food for the plant. During hot weather you'll need to ensure that the pots are regularly watered. Although drought resistant, grown in pots, Lavender needs moist soil – don't allow the pots to dry out completely at any time. During the winter the biggest danger is from too much water; although frost resistant it may be necessary to bring Lavender pots indoors – or into an unheated greenhouse to offer extra protection. If keeping Lavender outdoors, check regularly to ensure that the soil is not waterlogged – move the plants to a sheltered position by a wall to reduce the amount of rain falling on them if necessary.

Lavender grows relatively slowly but can become wild and bushy if not kept under control. Experts vary in their opinion as to when is the best time to prune lavender but all agree that regular pruning will keep the plant neat, trim and compact. Pruning should be done before or after flowering – so spring or autumn are the two times that are generally recommended. Many professional growers would argue that Lavender should be pruned back in autumn. Simply use secateurs to remove the stalks and some of the current years growth leaving some greenery at the base of the plant.

Lavender

Propagating new Lavender plants is remarkably easy – you can take green cuttings of softwood (stalks that have yet to become woody) at the start of the growing season in early summer. Cuttings from the hardwood of the Lavender will also root well but need to be taken at the end of the season – in late summer or during the autumn. These cuttings will be best established inside – either in a greenhouse, porch or well-lit window. Seeds can also be gathered from the flowers – simply remove the flowers in late summer and dry.

Harvesting Lavender

Cultivating Lavender for harvesting is a little like coppicing wood; newly established plants will only put out a small number of shoots in their first year. You should trim these before they flower in order to encourage more (and fuller) growth. In its second year the plant should double in size and you can harvest the lavender – the plant may only produce two or three bunches in this year. By the third year you'll find that the plant has grown yet again – by about two thirds, depending on your local climate. From this point on, correctly harvested, the plant will continue to produce an abundant crop each year. In most cases, well cared for, Lavender will live and produce good crops for upwards of twenty years.

If you are growing lavender for use in cooking, or in herbal remedies, the best time to harvest is just before the flowers open, when the buds are fully formed. This will capture the best scent/flavor and will contain the highest ratio of essential oil. Scent/flavor will fade once the plants have flowered and the later you harvest, the lower the potency of the herb. Harvested just before flowering will also make the buds easier to detach from the stalk once the plant is dried. We'll look in more detail at drying or extracting oil from the plant later in this book but drying can be completed outdoors if the weather is appropriate or indoors (filling your home with a strong, beautiful scent).

Chapter 3

Lavender for Healing

Research into the properties and uses of Lavender have confirmed to some extent that the traditional "folklore" uses of the plant have some sound scientific basis. Lavender has been shown to have a calming, soothing effect and inhaling the scent has been found to have a sedative effect. While science has confirmed what many traditional healers have long held to be true there is more research needed on the potential benefits of the plant. It is, however, considered by herbalists to be one of the most powerful herbal remedies available. Both the dried flowers and essential oil are used in preparing herbal treatments.

Lavender is believed to be useful at treating the following injuries and conditions;

- anxiety
- aches and pains
- bites, scratches and minor burns.
- Eczema and acne
- coughs, colds and congestion

Ashley Stone

- depression
- dizziness
- fevers
- fatigue
- headaches
- insomnia
- stress
- sunburn

Lavender

Lavender is rich in several molecules which help to explain its beneficial qualities. It contains high levels of "esters" which have calming and anti-spasmodic qualities. Other molecules that the plant contains have strong anti-bacterial and anti-inflammatory qualities. The oil produced from Lavender has the following properties:

- Antidepressant
- Analgesic
- Antiseptic
- Cicatrizant (meaning that it promotes the formation of scar tissue)
- Expectorant (this induces the body to increase fluid secretion thereby clearing the respiratory tract)
- Vulnerary (curative of wounds).

Lavender oil can be distilled at home (we'll cover the basic process later in this book) but can easily be bought and is considered an essential ingredient in many a household First Aid cabinet. To make the most of the benefits of Lavender oil the following methods can be used to address a number of conditions or injuries.

Muscle Strain Relief

For relieving tired, aching muscles (or to reduce stress) a hot, Lavender bath can't be beaten! Add up to 8 drops of lavender essential oil as you are running the bath and for extra luxury add Lavender bath salts or half a cup of milk (this will help to disperse the oil thoroughly through the water). For a quick stress relieving shower, add 3 drops of oil to a small cap-full of water and pour this over your head and rinse off. You can also add Lavender oil to your shampoo for effective cleaning and to relax neck muscles.

Coughs, Colds and Chest Problems

To help relieve colds, coughs and breathing problems, infusing the air in your home with Lavender is a simple, effective method. Use an oil burner and add 6-8 drops of essential oil – you can mix this with water in the vaporizer. Top up from time to time as the scent begins to fade. In addition – for fast relief – simply add 2-3 drops to a tissue and inhale immediately. This will help to clear blocked sinuses and encourage your body to produce more fluid which then aids in clearing mucus from blocked airways. For the worst colds and coughs inhale lavender steam. Add 4-6 drops of essential oil to a bowl of piping hot water, lean over this and cover your head and the bowl with a towel, inhale deeply and repeat several times a day.

Skin Conditions and Acne

For eczema, acne or dry skin conditions the steam inhalation method above has been noted to be highly effective. The antibacterial qualities in Lavender are believed to reduce the bacteria in the skin which cause pimples and blackheads that are a feature of acne. Again, the oils increase hydration by encouraging the body to produce fluids and this can make the inhalation effective for many skin conditions as well as those mentioned above.

Sprains and Strains

For sprains and strains a Lavender oil massage is an excellent way to find fast relief. You should mix the essential oil with a carrier oil (vegetable oil can be used but almond or lightly scented oils are best). The anti-inflammatory qualities of the lavender oil will help to relieve the pain and the oil will also enter the bloodstream through the skin, aiding relaxation and further pain relief.

Stings and Scratches

A simple Lavender compress can be created to treat bites, minor burns, stings or scratches. This will reduce inflammation and soreness very quickly and has been used medicinally for much of our history. Simply add around 8 drops of Lavender oil to a small bowl and fill with hot water. Stir this for a few minutes and add a cloth or bandage allowing the oil and water to soak into it. You can then apply the bandage/cloth to the affected area.

Burns and Sunburn

Minor burns or scalds will be eased using Lavender oil but only treat small burns in this way. Always seek medical advice for a more serious burn. To treat a minor burn (including sunburn) with Lavender simply massage a drop or two of pure lavender oil onto the affected part of the body. Avoid using pure oil on broken skin, however.

Alopecia Areata

Yet to be fully researched, Lavender appears to have a beneficial affect on those suffering from hair loss caused by this autoimmune disease. Massage several drops onto the scalp daily – this can be necessary for six to eight months. In many cases the regrowth of hair has been noted to be thicker when lavender oil is used than with other essential oils.

Dried Lavender Uses

Lavender tea is not only extremely delicious but it's been proven time and again to help relieve stress and anxiety. A few dried buds added to boiling water and steeped for a couple of minutes will help to calm nerves and settle anxious minds. A good mixture is Chamomile and Lavender – both herbs have excellent stress relief qualities.

Simply adding a bunch of dried lavender to any room will help to spread the fragrant scent around your home. Additionally you can create home-made candles using dried lavender buds. Add these to heated wax along with essential oil for extra fragrance.

Dried lavender can be used to make Lavender sachets – simply sew a small muslin bag and fill with buds. These make great small gifts and can be placed under (or on) your pillow to aid healthy, deep sleep. If you suffer from severe insomnia it's worth harvesting a large quantity and creating a larger pillow. Lavender/chamomile tea just before bedtime should also help.

Hang bunches of dried lavender in closets and drawers; this will add a little scent but is also believed to keep moths and bugs out of clothing.

Lavender Salve

Lavender salve is easy to make and can be used to treat cuts, burns and sores. It is also a great lip balm for dry, chapped lips and is even a great home-made insect repellent.

Heat up half a cup of olive/almond or ground nut oil in a pan and add a cup full of dried lavender flowers. Stir over a low heat for about ten minutes and then leave to cool for twenty.

Fill a pan with about an inch of water and heat, add a cup to the pan and 2 tablespoons of grated beeswax. You can add vitamin E to the mixture – just use the contents of a capsule – and stir until the wax is melted. Add the infused lavender oil and stir until everything is mixed well.

Pour into a jar and cool; store in a dark place once sealed. Add 10 drops of essential oil for extra scent and effectiveness.

Safety Notes

Lavender has been used for centuries to relieve and cure many conditions. Like all herbs it has many beneficial qualities but there may be some side-effects for some users. It's important to seek professional medical advice if you have any concerns but the main potential side-effects that should be considered are noted below.

Interactions with antidepressants

Lavender does promote relaxation but if you are using central nervous depressants this can make their effects stronger. These include morphine (for pain relief) and a range of anti-depressants, check with your doctor if you are taking any of this type of medication.

Allergic Reactions

A very small number of people may experience an allergic reaction to Lavender based oils, cosmetics and soaps. Again, check with your doctor if you are concerned before using Lavender.

Pregnant and Breastfeeding Women

Lavender is not normally recommended for women who are pregnant or while breastfeeding. Always check with a midwife or medical professional before using any medications (herbal or otherwise) if you are pregnant or are breastfeeding your baby.

Children and Lavender

Generally, Lavender in oral form is not recommended for children. Oils can be used, but prolonged use of Lavender oil has been suggested as a cause of "gynecomastia" (breast development in males) in young boys. Although no firm evidence has yet been studied on lavender's relation to this condition, many parents prefer not to treat children with lavender based products.

Chapter 4

Preserving Lavender

Given that it has so many beneficial qualities it's likely that you'll be keen to grow large quantities (space permitting) and harvest equally large quantities each year. While Lavender does keep very well in dried form it will lose some of its potency over time. Storing and using a crop of lavender for later is relatively simple. The main ways to store your abundant crop are; drying, distilling and infusing oil. In this chapter we'll look at all three options and the advantages and disadvantages of each.

Drying Lavender

Drying is the simplest way to preserve Lavender and also offers a range of options for using it for both scent and medicinal purposes. When harvesting cut the stems close to the ground to leave a good long stalk. Bunch the individual stalks together in bunches of around one hundred stems. Tie these close to the end of the stalk with either string or a rubber band and then hang the bunches upside down. For best results (in terms of color and scent preservation) hang the bunches in a warm, dark and dry location indoors.

Lavender

You can dry lavender in this way in a green house but exposure to sunlight may bleach some of the color during the drying process. If you choose this method try placing the bunches in a loose fitting paper bag – this protects them from direct sunlight. Pierce holes in the bags to allow a good circulation of air. Lavender can also be dried outdoors in the air – as long as it will not risk getting wet. Again, this may bleach some of the color and scent from the Lavender.

You can also oven dry Lavender by placing in bunches in the oven at 180 degrees Fahrenheit (80 degrees Celsius), this will take approximately four to six hours but may be costly if you have large quantities to dry!

Drying Lavender is the simplest way to preserve it; the Lavender dried in this manner will last for several years, although fragrance and color will both reduce over time. You can revitalize the scent by simply squeezing the bunch.

The main advantage to drying Lavender is that it is so simple that anybody should be able to do it. Although it can take a few weeks to dry there's very little work involved. The main disadvantage of drying is that (if you have large quantiles) the finished product will take up a reasonable amount of space and, as mentioned above, color and potency of scent will deteriorate over time. Dried Lavender can be used to make teas, pillows, simply added to a bath and added to potpourri or hung in a room to decorate and add a gentle, relaxing scent.

Distilling Lavender Essential Oil

OK, so essential oils are fairly easy to come by these days so distilling your own may sound like hard work! However, if you have a large harvest to deal with you may well want to give home-distilling a try! Small home distillation kits can also be readily purchased so even if you don't intend to farm Lavender on a grand scale this is still a feasible option – and it's also a truly satisfying way to stock up on your own, home-grown and distilled essential oil.

Distillation works by extracting essential oils by effectively stewing/boiling the raw material – Lavender in this case – and passing the steam given off through a 'condenser'. This is basically a tube! You can create your own distilling kit but, in most cases, it will make sense to buy a small, home distilling kit. These are widely available on-line and many are designed for distilling smaller quantiles of essential oil. There are three main methods – water, steam and alcohol extraction.

Water based distillation simply involves soaking the Lavender in water for around 24 – 48 hours. Once this has been completed the flowers should be strained from the liquid and this is then boiled in the condenser to produce the oil.

Steam based is similar but in this case the water and Lavender are separated; the water is boiled and steam passes through the Lavender, extracting the essential oils – the steam flows through the condenser and you are left with Lavender essential oil.

Alcohol extraction is very much the same as water based but instead of soaking in water you'll need alcohol of around 50% volume. Again, the Lavender is soaked for up to 48 hours and then the strained liquid needs to be boiled to extract the oils.

Generally, for Lavender, the steam and alcohol based methods will produce the highest quality oils. As mentioned small, domestic stills can be purchased to be used in all three methods.

Compared to simply drying, distilling allows you to process larger quantities of Lavender and the oil produced will store indefinitely. It also has the advantage of having a wider range of uses – if you dry and distill Lavender you can take full advantage of all of the different uses mentioned in this book.

The main disadvantage with distilling is that it may cost a little more in terms of initial outlay for equipment. Distilling is also a slow, relatively labor intensive process and takes does require some skill. For those with smaller quantities of Lavender distilling may not be the best option but it can certainly be a good way to make the most of your Lavender crop if you have larger amounts.

Infused Lavender Oil

This is an alternative method to store and make use of your Lavender and is a simple way to store the best of the scent from Lavender! Infused oil can be used in cooking, for massage and can also be used in scent burners – although it is not as potent as distilled essential oil. Infusing means just that, and the process simply captures the scent of Lavender rather than the essential oil.

To infuse Lavender you'll need a carrier oil. Any food-grade oil will do but those with limited scent and flavor of their own will be best suited. Almond, sunflower or Ground Nut Oil are good options. The latter, in particular, has little scent or flavor of its own so may be the best choice.

Add Lavender flowers to a jar with a seal-able, tight fitting lid. Pour your oil over the flowers – use a ratio of approximately 1/3 Lavender to 2/3 oil. Place this in a warm, but dark, place and leave for anything from 48 hours to two weeks. The longer you store the oil like this the stronger the scent/flavor will be in the finished oil. Shake or turn the jar

Lavender

at least once a day. If you're only storing for a few days do this several times a day.

When this process is completed you will need to strain out the Lavender flowers to create the finished oil. Store the oil in a sealed bottle, or jar, again in a dark place, and use as required. The oil should last for up to a year – possibly longer.

Infused oil has a wide range of uses and can be used with or instead of essential oil for many of the applications in this book. It is a simple process that anybody can complete. Unlike drying it preserves the scent very well for longer periods, if stored correctly, and unlike distilling does not need any complicated equipment. Apart from preparation time and a little shaking every now and then it is not a labor intensive method.

Disadvantages – are few! Infused oil is a great alternative to distilling your own essential oil but it does not have the potency of distilled oil. However, it can be combined with commercially sourced essential oil and it's an option for harvesting and storing that will be suitable for many people.

Chapter 5

Cooking with Lavender

Today, many of us think of Lavender as an attractive plant that can be found in country gardens or as a decorative plant for borders in many settings. Traditionally it was found in many herb gardens and, as member of the mint family, the plant is technically a herb. For much of its history, Lavender place in herb gardens was not simply to keep away unwanted insects (and attract pollen spreading ones). Although both of these factors played a part Lavender's presence in herb gardens it was not simply decorative. Lavender has been used in cookery for centuries and was a popular addition to any number of dishes throughout history – prized for its floral scent and slightly sweet taste.

The sweet taste should be a clue to Lavenders many culinary uses. It is commonly found in many recipes for sweets and confectionery. However, culinary uses aren't limited to sweets and Lavender can be found flavoring soups, stews and savory dishes in many historic cook books. If you've fallen in love with Lavender as a garden plant, in this chapter we'll look at some recipes that may well have you falling in love with Lavender in the kitchen as well.

Before we get to the recipes there are some simple rules to follow when cooking with Lavender. The first is that a *little* Lavender goes a long way! Lavender is highly scented and using too much will result in a highly perfumed (possibly inedible) dish. Large amounts of Lavender will also tend to make a dish bitter and, again, distinctly unpalatable! The second point to remember is that in the recipes in this book you should use fresh Lavender if possible but where this is not available substitute 1/3 of the quantity of dried flowers.

Simple Lavender Cookery Tricks

Lavender can be added to salads for extra color and a gentle floral flavor. Remember a little Lavender goes a long way, the lightest sprinkling will do.

Where any recipe calls for herbs (most do) consider substituting Lavender. Particularly successful options will include breads; instead of rosemary, for example, use a little Lavender instead.

Lavender sugar is easy to create and is a perfect topping for cakes and cookies. Add flowers to a jar of sugar and mix well, sealing and storing for several weeks. The sugar, minus the flowers, can be sprinkled over the top of the finished cake or cookie.

Savory Lavender Cooking

Smoked Salmon with Lavender and Dill.

This is a delicious and surprising dish. Simply wrap smoked salmon fillets in foil, with half a head of Lavender each – crumple the individual flowers over each fillet of salmon. Sprinkle with a similar amount of dill, add salt and pepper to taste, add a knob of butter to each and wrap the foil lightly over the salmon creating a loose bag around each. Steam or bake in the oven for twenty minutes on a moderate heat.

Pork or Lamb with Lavender.

Both of these meats have a light sweet flavor which is complimented very well by the sweet, floral aroma of Lavender. Simple grilled chops can be transformed using this surprising herb. Use ½ teaspoon of dried Lavender and combine with salt and pepper to taste, 2 teaspoons of dried thyme and 1 teaspoon of chopped, fresh rosemary. Combine the herbs in a tablespoon of olive oil and rub this mixture over the chops until they are covered thoroughly. Wrap the chops in plastic and leave for 2 hours at room temperature. Grill on a medium heat for up to 5 minutes each side.

Wine and Lavender Sauce

This can be made to pour over any meat – red meats, in particular, work well with this sauce. Simply add one or two Lavender flowers to 1/3 of a bottle of red wine, season with a little salt and pepper and then bring to the boil. Simmer, covered over a moderate heat for twenty minutes and the turn the heat back up to reduce the sauce. Reduce until thick, stirring constantly. This can take a further twenty minutes depending on how thick you wish to have have the sauce.

Tuna Steaks with Lavender and Herb Crust

Combine a teaspoon of salt, 2 of black peppercorns, 2 teaspoons of fennel seeds, ½ teaspoon of Lavender flowers, 2-3 tablespoons of olive oil and 4 cups of savory mixed, fresh herbs of your choice in a mortar. Grind the herb mixture together gradually adding the oil. Once thoroughly mixed take your Tuna steaks and coat them liberally in the mixture. Heat a sauté pan to a high heat adding a teaspoon of oil and sear each side of the steaks for approximately 1 minute for a rare Tuna steak, a little longer if required. The Tuna can be served hot or refrigerated to serve with salad – refrigerate for no more than three hours to retain the full flavor.

Lavender Stews

Lavender can be added to just about most stews or casseroles to create a subtle, slightly sweet flavor. Simply substitute one of the herbs you would normally add (or the recipe you are using suggests); stews are great "winter warmers" and with the addition of Lavender they become a gentle, surprising reminder of warmer days! The trick is to be very careful with your amounts! For a stew to serve four portions add no more than a single flower head (whole). You can also use leaves – which will produce a much lighter, subtler flavor. Simply pick and wash a few fresh leaves from the plant and tear these a couple of times. Add to your stew once all other ingredients have been added or towards the end of cooking if using dried flowers/leaves.

Sweet Treats

Creme Brulee with Lavender

Creme brulee and Lavender were probably made for each other. The crunchy, but light, brulee works perfectly with the subtle flora flavor of Lavender flowers. Use 4 cups of thick cream, 1 tablespoon of dried lavender flowers, 8 egg yolks and ¾ cup of sugar.

Heat the oven to 300 degrees and butter six ramekins in advance. In a saucepan add the cream and lavender flowers on a medium heat allowing them to simmer for a few minutes. Remove from the heat and set aside for ten minutes, straining the flowers from the cream after this time. In a separate bowl gently whisk the egg yolks and ½ cup of sugar until creamy. Add the strained lavender cream mixture slowly to the yolk/sugar mixture. Divide this into the ramekins.

Lavender

The brulees should then be baked in a "bath" (a deep baking tray with enough hot water to come about half way up the sides of the ramekins) for about sixty minutes, or until the mixture has set at the edges but is still slightly loose in the center. Once cooked remove from the oven and leave to cool before refrigerating for 2 hours (minimum). Just before serving sprinkle with 2 teaspoons of sugar (Lavender sugar is, of course, ideal for this) and crisp with a hand-held torch. (You can grill for a few minutes if you don't have one of these).

Lavender Shortbread

Delicately sweet and deliciously refined, Lavender shortbread makes a perfect afternoon treat, or gift. It's also a gift that will surprise your friends and family with your skill!

You'll need; 1 ½ cups of softened butter, ¼ cup of confectioner's sugar; 2/3 cup of sugar (again, Lavender sugar is ideal), 2 tablespoons of finely chopped fresh Lavender, 1 tablespoon of chopped, fresh mint; 1 teaspoon of grated lemon zest, 2 ½ cups of flour; ½ cup of cornstarch, ¼ teaspoon of salt.

In a bowl, mix the butter, confectioner's sugar and plain sugar together until the mixture is light and fluffy. Add the lavender, mint and the lemon zest.

In a separate bowl, combine the flours and then gradually mix into the batter until thoroughly mixed. Divide this mixture into a couple of balls, wrap in plastic, flatten to about an inch thickness and chill in the refrigerator for an hour.

Setting the oven at 325 degrees, take the dough from the refrigerator and roll out on a lightly floured surface to ¼ of inch thickness, cut into shapes and place on a cookie sheet in the oven to bake for around 20 minutes. Cool for a moment or two then transfer to a cooling rack to completely cool.

Conclusion

Thank you again for buying this book!

I hope this book was able to help you find inspiration on the many and varied uses of Lavender. More than simply a decorative plant, Lavender has a great range of uses for both health and cookery.

The next step is to get out in the garden and start to cultivate your very own crop of this amazing herb!

Finally, if you enjoyed this book, please take the time to share your thoughts and post a review on Amazon. It'd be greatly appreciated!

Thank you and good luck!

Made in the USA
Monee, IL
02 April 2021